100 SURPRISING APPLE CIDER VINEGAR REMEDIES

By Emily Taylor

The information herein is offered for informational purposes solely, and is universal as so. The presentation of the information is without contract or any type of guarantee assurance.

The trademarks that are used are without any consent, and the publication of the trademark is without permission or backing by the trademark owner. All trademarks and brands within this book are for clarifying purposes only and are the owned by the owners themselves, not affiliated with this document.

Disclaimer and Terms of Use: The Author and Publisher has strived to be as accurate and complete as possible in the creation of this book, notwithstanding the fact that he does not warrant or represent at any time that the contents within are accurate due to the rapidly changing nature of the Internet. While all attempts have been made to verify information provided in this publication, the Author and Publisher assumes no responsibility for errors, omissions, or contrary interpretation of the subject matter herein.

Any perceived slights of specific persons, peoples, or organizations are unintentional. In practical advice books, like anything else in life, there are no guarantees of results. Readers are cautioned to rely on their own judgment about their individual circumstances and act accordingly.

This book is not intended for use as a source of legal, medical, business, accounting or financial advice. All readers are advised to seek services of competent professionals in the legal, medical, business, accounting, and finance fields.

TABLE OF CONTENTS

WHAT IS APPLE CIDER VINEGAR (ACV)?

Apple cider vinegar is a natural vinegar made by fermenting apples. It is commonly used as an essential ingredient in cooking, but over centuries it has also been proven to be an overall remedy and relief for various problems. May it be health problems, beauty problems or household problems, apple cider vinegar is known for its many uses and benefits.

WHEN DID IT START?

The use of apple cider vinegar started around 400 BC. It was first used by Hippocrates, The Father of Medicine, as a medicinal product for his remedial treatments. Hippocrates would recommend his patients drinking apple cider vinegar to as treatment for cough and colds. It was traditionally used by people for wound healing, cleaning and sanitizing, and food preservation. Apple cider vinegar has certainly come a long way from being a mere folk remedy to a reliable modern natural-made medicine.

TWO TYPES OF APPLE CIDER VINEGAR

• ORGANIC APPLE CIDER VINEGAR

The organic type of apple cider vinegar is made by naturally fermenting apples without the use of heat. It didn't undergo any type of artificial process and is not refined. Unlike commercial types of apple cider vinegar, the organic type is purely natural and appears a little cloudy because it contains the "mother" of vinegar. The "mother" refers to a colony of good bacteria. These bacteria are considered as the most beneficial part of this type of vinegar, is gut-friendly and the main source of apple cider vinegar's many benefits. Organic apple cider vinegar is also referred to as raw, unpasteurized or unfiltered apple cider vinegar.

• COMMERCIAL APPLE CIDER VINEGAR

This type of vinegar is made through a process called pasteurization. Since fermenting takes too much time, manufacturers opt to artificially create a fermented apple cider vinegar with the same ingredient but without consuming too much time. Pasteurization is done by heating filtered vinegar and removing sediments if there are any. Unlike the organic kind of apple cider vinegar, commercial apple cider vinegar has a clear or translucent appearance because the "mother" of vinegar has been taken out.

HOW RAW APPLE CIDER VINEGAR IS MADE

Apple cider vinegar is made from ripe, freshly crushed, apples that are fermented. It goes through a natural process without using heat. First, the crushed apples are exposed to yeast to start the alcoholic fermentation process. In this process, the sugars from the apple are turned into alcohol. Second, good bacteria is added to the alcohol solution which further ferments the alcohol and turns into acetic acid.

CHEMICAL COMPOSITION

Apple cider vinegar contains only 3 calories per tablespoon (15 grams) and practically no carbohydrates. It has minimum amounts of potassium, phosphorus, magnesium, and calcium. Because of the apple content, it may contain several minerals and vitamins like: vitamin C, vitamins B1, B2 and B6; biotin, folic acid, niacin, pectin, and pantothenic acid.

The acetic acid formed during fermentation is the main active compound which is responsible for apple cider vinegar's countless benefits. Apple cider vinegar also contains a generous amount of amino acids that are effective antiseptics and also work as antibiotics.

WHICH APPLE CIDER VINEGAR TO USE?

Use only organic, raw, unfiltered, unpasteurized apple cider vinegar that has the mother intact. All of this has to be written on the label. The mother is, again, the main reason for all its wonderful benefits, therefore it is essential. Make sure to shake it well before using to disperse the mother evenly.

CAUTION!

Apple cider vinegar is highly acidic. Acetic acid, its main active compound, might be harsh to consume for some. And when used as a remedy for skin ailments and infections, it may cause the skin to dry. To ease the acidic content of ACV, dilute it in water before consumption or for a much safer usage, consult your doctor.

BELOW ARE 100 SURPRISINGLY AND PROVEN EFFECTIVE USES OF APPLE CIDER VINEGAR.

1. SOOTHES A SORE THROAT

A sore throat is commonly caused by viral illnesses like colds. You may experience difficulty in swallowing and breathing, accompanied by a hoarseness in the voice which is very uncomfortable. The acid in apple cider vinegar will kill the bacteria that's in the throat area. The next time uneasiness occurs from a sore throat, grab a bottle of apple cider vinegar. Dissolve 1 tablespoon of apple cider vinegar and 1 teaspoon of salt in a glass of warm water and gargle. You can add honey or lemon juice to compensate for the taste. Drink several times a day as needed.

2. DIGESTIVE TONIC TO RELIEVE INDIGESTION

Indigestion may be a pain or discomfort in the upper abdomen (dyspepsia) and symptoms usually appear after eating and drinking. Apple cider vinegar helps digestion by increasing stomach acid. For immediate relief from digestive problems, mix 1-3 tablespoons of apple cider vinegar in a glass of water and consumes 10 to 15 minutes before meals. This will greatly improve digestion and nutrient assimilation by increasing HCI production. For those who have excessive stomach acid, since apple cider vinegar contains an ample amount of acid too, opt for adding a small amount of baking soda in your tonic to neutralize the acidity.

3. LOWERS CHOLESTEROL AND LOWERS RISK OF HEART DISEASE

One of the most common causes of deaths is heart disease. A disturbing increase in bad cholesterol may also increase the risk of a heart attack. Studies showed that apple cider lowers HDL and triglyceride levels. Apple cider also contains chlorogenic acid which protects LDL cholesterol from becoming oxidized. Dilute at least 1-2 tablespoon (15-30mL) of apple cider vinegar in warm water per day to help regulate cholesterol levels in the body.

4. AIDS IN WEIGHT LOSS

Obesity is one factor that results from common illnesses such as heart disease and diabetes. Several studies suggest that drinking apple cider vinegar can increase satiety, helping you eat much less which should eventually lead to losing pounds of weight. Apple cider vinegar together with a high carb intake increase feeling of fullness, thus resulting in lesser calorie intake. A study conducted in obese individuals show that daily consumption of apple cider vinegar led to reduced belly fat and lost pounds of 2.6 from 15 mL of continuous apple cider consumption for 12 weeks. Imagine the effect when workout and daily exercises in incorporated into your daily routine; weight loss would be a piece of cake.

5. CLEARS STUFFY NOSE

Colds and flu are caused by viral infections characterized by a stuffy nose and constant coughing which often occur during changes in temperature or because of a weak immune system. Apple cider vinegar contains potassium that eventually thins mucus and acetic acid that kills bacteria formation, which greatly contributes to nasal congestion. For immediate relief, mix 1-3 tablespoon of apple cider in a glass of water and drink, especially in the morning, 30 minutes before breakfast, to help sinus drainage.

6. LOWERS BLOOD SUGAR LEVELS

One study shows that apple cider vinegar can help stimulate digestive enzymes and inhibit some of these. This will slow the breakdown of carbohydrates into sugar and gives the body enough time to pull it out of the bloodstream thus preventing sugar levels from spiking. People who have diabetes would opt to drink a glass of water with one to two tablespoons of apple cider vinegar in the morning before breakfast to inhibit digestive enzymes and regulate blood sugar levels.

7. DERMATITIS (ECZEMA) RELIEF

Dermatitis is a skin condition resulting from direct irritation of the skin from outside factors or allergies and is characterized by redness, swelling, and small blisters on the skin. It is also called eczema. Itchiness may result if the condition is short-term, while the skin may become thick and crusty if the condition is long-term.

Apple cider can help sanitize the inflamed area of the skin, reduce inflammation and prompt healing. Add honey and apple cider vinegar (measurement depends upon the needs and the broadness of the affected skin area) then apply this mixture once a day to the inflamed area. If immediate relief is not attained, better yet consult a professional.

8. ACHES AND PAIN RELIEF

Muscle and joint pains are commonly related to arthritis. The acetic acid in apple cider vinegar helps with the absorption of calcium in the body, resulting to better bone and joint conditions. Add 1 tablespoon of apple cider vinegar in a glass of water or in your daily herbal tea and add honey to sweeten the drink. Significant changes can be observed in just a few weeks.

9. IMPROVE INSULIN SENSITIVITY

People who have type 2 diabetes often lose their sensitivity to insulin. This results in an increase in blood sugar levels since the hormone, insulin stops signaling cells to remove sugar from the blood. One study suggested that continuous consumption of apple cider vinegar improved insulin sensitivity in about 19 percent of individuals with type 2 diabetes and 34 of those with pre-diabetes. Make it a habit to drink 2 tablespoons of apple cider vinegar before bedtime.

10. ENERGY BOOST

Fatigue occurs when the body is pushed to the limit. Everyday work could cause stress and ultimately lead to fatigue or worse. Regular intake of supplements in addition to a well-balanced diet could help relieve fatigue but there are ways of further boosting this.

Apple cider vinegar helps fight fatigue with its potassium content and enzymes. Enzymes help in the breakdown of carbohydrates we intake thus giving the body the sufficient energy it needs. Apple cider vinegar also contains amino acids that help prevent lactic acid buildup in your body and further prevent fatigue.

11. DETOXIFY BODY

Every single day, even without us knowing, we actually take in numerous toxins. This is why there's a need for regular detoxification. The most common way is by consuming detoxifying drinks. There are a lot of other ingredients you can incorporate into your detox drink including: lemon juice, ground ginger, cinnamon, honey, cayenne pepper, etc. Below is a suggested recipe for detox tea using apple cider vinegar.

- 1 cup warm water

- 2 tbsp ACV

- 2 tbsp lemon juice

- 1 tbsp raw honey

- 1 tsp cinnamon

- Dash of cayenne

12. TREATS ACID REFLUX AND HEARTBURN

Acid reflux is characterized by a burning sensation in the upper chest and throat area from the acid that forms in the stomach. Apple cider vinegar helps in balancing stomach pH by neutralizing stomach acid. It is advised to mix 2 tablespoons of apple cider in 200mL of water for treating acid reflux. For a more effective and immediate result, try adding ¼ teaspoon of baking soda. Baking soda, as well, mitigates the pH level of acid and restores acid-alkaline balance in the stomach.

13. KILLS CANDIDA

Candida is the most common type of yeast infection. This fungus is usually found in the mouth, intestinal tract and vagina, and results from overgrowth of yeast in the body. It is hard to treat since it affects the infected person in different ways, depending on their hygiene and immune system condition.

ACV is one of nature's strongest antibiotics. It can kill the bacteria, virus and protozoa for a relief from yeast infection. The acetic acid in ACV helps lower the vagina's pH level and makes it less tolerable from yeast infection. Apple cider can be used as a mouthwash, a drink, as a soak or as a body bath. Mix two tablespoons of apple cider vinegar in a bottle or glass of water. Apply to infected area or drink as needed.

14. JELLY FISH STING REMEDY

Jellyfish stings are painful and itchy at the same time. Rashes may also appear and if not treated abruptly, progressive effects like nausea, vomiting, abdominal pain, muscle spasm, etc. could occur. The sooner the sting is treated, the better. Pour apple cider vinegar directly on to the affected area. The acid from ACV will immediately prevent the venom from spreading to other parts of the body and eliminate other bacteria that may cause infections. It will also get rid of the itches.

15. REGULATES BODY PH

The optimal pH is in between 7.3 to 7.4 for humans. The moment one's pH goes outside that range, the more one's metabolism malfunctions and worse, stop working. Once apple cider vinegar is in the body and is broken down by enzymes, it promotes alkalinity. Make it a habit to drink a mixture of apple cider vinegar and water daily to balance body pH.

16. RELIEVES PMS

Bloating, cramping, cravings, headaches and irritability are just some PMS symptoms ladies undergo every month and proves to be frustrating and absolutely a hassle. There are women who attest to the fact that their PMS has lessened with this natural remedy. Apple cider vinegar helps reduce period muscle cramps by easing the uterus muscles. Apple cider helps reduce the overall duration of ladies' menstrual cycle as well as reducing the amounts of blood you lose from your body. Mix 1 to 2 tablespoons of raw apple cider vinegar in a glass of water.

17. TREATS URINARY TRACT INFECTION

Urinary tract infection is an infection that affects parts of the urinary system including the kidney, uterus, urethra and urinary bladder. Apple cider vinegar is rich in potassium and enzymes that can help eliminate and prevent bacteria from spreading and causing urinary tract infection. Constant intake of apple cider vinegar may prevent a lot of infections and diseases from transpiring including UTI. However, it may be a problem to treat UTI with ACV once the person is already infected. Nevertheless, you can still try by mixing 1-2 tablespoons of apple cider vinegar in a glass of water and drink.

18. DISSOLVE KIDNEY STONES

Kidney stones are hard, stone-like and crystalline minerals formed in the kidney due to the ingredients of food that we intake. These are kidney stones that are too small to create any changes in the body, but there are ones that may result in severe pain in the abdomen and can cause blood in the urine. Drinking apple cider vinegar will greatly help remove and dissolve kidney stones. Drink 1 tbsp of apple cider vinegar mixed with a glass of water throughout the day especially before meal times.

19. KILLS CANCER CELLS OR SLOW THEIR GROWTH

A lot of studies are ongoing for considering apple cider vinegar as a natural treatment to cancer. With the many health benefits of apple cider vinegar, it would be likely to slow cancer cells growth or maybe kill cancer cells completely. Some researchers and nutritionists believe that maintaining the proper alkaline and acid balance in one's system will help prevent cancer, and apple cider vinegar can do just that. Continue drinking diluted apple cider vinegar each morning to help the body attain alkaline stage and restore natural body pH.

20. IMMUNE BOOSTING

One's immune system is important for fighting bad bacteria and preventing viruses, that may result in the flu or greater, from spreading to the other parts of the body. Apple cider vinegar contains healthy bacteria that helps the immune system fight off bad bacteria, thus preventing the body from many sickness-causing viruses to enter.

- 1 teaspoon apple cider vinegar

- 1 cup green tea

- A squeeze of lemon juice

- A drop or two of raw honey

- 1 small slice of ginger, crushed

- A dash of cinnamon

Steep the tea in water for 2-3 minutes. Remove the tea and add the remaining ingredients. The longer the ginger steeps, the stronger the drink will be. Stir well then remove the ginger slice before drinking.

21. RELIEVE DIARRHEA

Diarrhea is caused by a bacterial infection that causes intestinal spasm and makes you go to the bathroom countless times in a day. Apple cider vinegar could help in relieving diarrhea with its antibiotic properties. This will kill living bacteria and prevent it further spreading. Also, some experts say that apple cider vinegar contains enough amount of pectin, which helps increase the growth of good bacteria in the gut and can soothe intestinal spasms and inflammation. Mix 1 cup apple cider vinegar in 2 cups water and drink. There will be an automatic relief from diarrhea after intake.

22. SINUS PRESSURE RELIEF

Sinus infection causes inflammation or swelling in the lining of the sinuses. It is very annoying and uncomfortable and also leads to headaches. Finally, apple cider can help relieve sinus pressure by these simple ingredients found at home:

- ½ to 1 teaspoon apple cider vinegar

- 1 cup warm filtered water

Add apple cider vinegar to a cup of warm unfiltered water and stir well. Place an ample amount of the mixture on your palms and snort it up one nostril at a time.

23. WOUND DISINFECTANT (LOCAL ANTISEPTIC)

Apple cider vinegar has been used for treating wounds for centuries. Even the Father of Medicine, Hippocrates, used this as a means for treating his patients. Apple cider vinegar contains a generous amount of amino acids that are effective antiseptics and disinfectants. The acetic acid in apple cider also kills the bacteria and prevents buildup so that wounds would be free from any infections that may pass through the skin opening. Dilute 1 part apple cider vinegar in 2 parts water and use a cotton ball in applying the solution to the opening of the wound. Make sure you do this with clean hands.

24. DETOXIFY LIVER

Apple cider vinegar has natural detoxifying agents. It will help detox and cleanse the liver and at the same time is a great kick start for your mornings.

- 1 tablespoon apple cider vinegar

- 1 teaspoon lemon juice

- 1 teaspoon honey

- 1 glass water

Pour all the ingredients in the glass of water. Drink this early in the morning, 30 minutes before breakfast. Keep drinking ample water during your detox to prevent dehydration.

25. IMPROVE BONE HEALTH

Osteoporosis is a bone disease that develops as we age. Signs suggesting osteoporosis include loss of height, a curved upper back, back pain and broken bones. This may be caused by genetics, aging, nutrition and lifestyle. Apple cider vinegar contains calcium that helps in bone health. It also contains enzymes which are effective for breaking down food and increasing the release of calcium found in many of the foods we consume. Add two table spoons of apple cider vinegar to a glass of water and drink once each morning.

26. NAUSEA RELIEF

Nausea is typically caused by motion sickness, dizziness, fainting, etc. Apple cider vinegar can help in regulating blood flow, calming nerves and relaxing muscles to relieve the effects of nausea. Mix 1 tablespoon of apple cider vinegar with 1 cup of filtered water and drink when experiencing nausea. An alternative way is to add a tablespoon of apple cider vinegar in a cup of hot tea. The tea will help you relax and calm your insides.

27. STOP HICCUPS

One primary cause of hiccups is low stomach acid, thus drinking apple cider vinegar can help relieve it as well. Take a spoonful of apple cider vinegar and drink it. If the taste is a little too tarty for you, you can opt to dissolve the apple cider vinegar in a cup of water, mix it well and drink that instead. The sour taste in it will create a distraction and ultimately stop hiccups.

28. TREAT CRAMPS

Apple cider vinegar contains two important minerals: potassium and calcium. Low levels of potassium and calcium can often be the cause of cramps. An increased intake of calcium and potassium help will relax the muscles thus relieving cramps. Dilute 1 part apple cider vinegar in 2 parts water and add a teaspoon of honey to relive or even prevent nighttime cramp attacks. You can also add fruit juice to sweeten the taste.

29. BREAK A FEVER

While a fever leaves a person feeling weak and disoriented, this is also a good sign that one's immune system is working. It shows that there's a virus in our system, but the body is healthy enough to begin taking action against it. To reduce the symptoms of a fever, however, take 1 part apple cider vinegar and mix this with 2 parts cold water. Soak a cotton ball into the mixture and place this on the soles of your feet. Cover it with socks or plastic bags and leave it overnight. You can also soak a washcloth into the mixture and place them on your forehead.

30. SPRAIN COMPRESS

Before refrigerators were invented to make ice cubes used for relieving a sprained ankle, people used apple cider vinegar. Apple cider vinegar is best for blood circulation, thus it helps blood in the sprained part to flow freely and relieve it of the pain. There are numerous ways and procedures for using apple cider vinegar to treat sprains. The easiest and less hassle to do is by taking a piece of brown paper and soaking it properly with apple cider vinegar. Place this wet bag on the area of your sprained ankle. Immediate relief from pain will occur. If not, repeat the steps until the pain from the sprained ankle is relieved.

31. TREATING THE EFFECTS OF POISON IVY

Poison ivy is a plant that can produce rashes upon direct contact with the skin. The itchy rash doesn't start to show up until 12 to 72 hours after skin contact. Apple cider vinegar can help draw out the toxins in the rash, accelerate healing and reduce discomfort in no time. Use a brown paper bag and soak this in apple cider vinegar. Pat, it directly onto affected area. Leave it on the skin for several minutes and repeat of desired effect is not achieved yet. This is also to re-live oneself of the itch.

32. NUTRIENT ABSORPTION BOOSTER (ESPECIALLY IRON)

No matter how healthy and nutrient-filled the food that you eat might be, if the nutrients in those aren't absorbed completely by the body, it's a total loss. Proper stomach acid levels enable the body to absorb nutrients properly. Apple cider vinegar can aid in the absorption of nutrients from food that we eat by regulating stomach acid. It can also boost metabolism, which results in proper nutrient absorption. Consumption of apple cider vinegar will also increase the surface cells of the small intestine, therefore improving absorption of nutrients. Dilute one part apple cider vinegar with 2 parts water and drink in every morning to condition metabolism and stomach acid.

33. WARTS REMOVAL

Warts are skin infections which appear out of the blue. But the truth is, warts come from a virus that you may have acquired or come into contact with a few months before it appeared on your skin. Apple cider vinegar's acidic state causes the wart to soften and peel off from the skin naturally Apply a generous amount of petroleum jelly on warts and on the skin surrounding to prevent the burning sensation that happens when using apple cider vinegar directly. Mix 2 cups of apple cider vinegar in 1 cup of water, soak a cotton ball into mixture and apply directly to warts.

34. SOOTHES SUNBURN

We can't always escape the harsh heat of the sun especially during the summer season. In case you forget to put on sun block before basking under the sun for a long period of time, here is a natural, alternative way of treating sun burns overnight. You only need raw apple cider vinegar and organic coconut oil. Use a clean washcloth and soak it in cold water. Splash apple cider vinegar on the washcloth and apply to the affected area. Wait for a few minutes to let dry. Right after, rub some coconut oil on the sunburned area.

35. NATURAL DEODORANT

It's completely natural to have body odor. It's a way for the skin to eliminate toxins in the body through the pores. What isn't natural is to have smelly body odor and leave it there stinking. The use of antiperspirants and deodorants will find one way or another worsen the case rather than relieve it because of the chemical properties found in these. Using apple cider vinegar as a natural deodorant will kill the bacteria causing stinking body odor and preventing that bacteria to spread. Soak a cotton ball in water and apple cider vinegar mixture and apply directly on certain areas of the body. Do this once a week or more depending on the amount of bacteria present.

36. REMOVE MOLES

For some people, moles are additions to one's beauty. But recent studies show that moles which continuously grow in size can become a target for cancer cells. So, it's better to remove them early on. With the acetic content and anti-inflammatory properties in apple cider vinegar, it can help in effectively removing moles and prevent bacterial infections. For mole removal, you'll need a cotton ball, band-aid and apple cider vinegar. Dip the cotton ball in apple cider vinegar, apply on the mole and leave it there for 8 hours secured with a band-aid. Repeat this routine every day until the mole freely scabs up from the skin.

37. REDUCE ITCH FROM BUG BITES

Bug bites cause itchiness and swollen skin which can be very irritating and frustrating at the same time. There are a lot of remedies out there and using apple cider vinegar is one of them. The acid in apple cider vinegar will nix the itch and help in healing the bug bite. Mix 1 part of apple cider vinegar with equal parts of water and apply to this to the affected area. Remember to always dilute ACV before use as direct contact with the skin may cause irritation.

38. STOP OILY HAIR

While oil is good for the hair to stay healthy and frizz-free, excessive oil in the hair will leave hair prone to more dirt and bacteria. Dry hair will only need a minimum amount of apple cider vinegar, while those with oily hair would need more. By using apple cider vinegar, pH level in scalp will be balanced thus hair roots won't excrete too much oil. Mix 3 tablespoons or apple cider vinegar with a cup of water. Apply evenly to hair and leave for a couple of minutes. Rinse after.

39. CELLULITE CLEANSER

You can now skip those expensive cellulite treatments with just one homemade substitute. The acid and other components in apple cider vinegar help remove excess fat and other toxins. To get rid of unwanted cellulite, mix the following:

- 1 part apple cider vinegar

- 2 parts water

- 1 tsp honey

Apply this mixture on the area where you have cellulite and leave it for half an hour. Cleanse with warm water after. Note: Even if you faithfully apply this every day, it will only do a minimum effect without the help of daily exercise and a well-balanced diet.

40. FADE BRUISES

When it comes to bruises, apple cider vinegar is proven to help increase the blood flow near the bruised part of the skin, thus dissipating pooled blood around the bruised area. This eventually lessens the greenish color formed on the skin and fades the bruise. Mix equal parts of apple cider vinegar and water. Soak a cotton ball into the mixture and apply on the bruised area for about half an hour. You can fasten it the cotton ball with a band-aid or a gauze.

41. FACIAL TONER

Skip the expensive store-bought facial toners that you use every day and try this homemade facial toner. It is easy to make and has so many benefits on the skin. Applying apple cider vinegar on the face, with other equally beneficial ingredients, will balance the natural pH of the skin, eliminate dead skin cells, clears excess oil and leaves skin soft and refreshed.

- 1 cup apple cider vinegar

- Filtered water

- ¼ cup honey

- 2-3 drops essential oils

Mix the ingredients together and store this in a plastic container. Use a cotton ball to apply the mixture on the face while avoiding the space near the eyes. You can also store the mixture in a spray bottle and spray onto the face to freshen up. You can opt to cleanse after usage or not.

42. MAKEUP REMOVER

It is important to remove makeup after a whole day of wearing them to prevent damaging the skin. Not doing so may cause skin infection and breakouts. There are so many makeup removers that can be bought from stores but you can also try a natural alternative by using apple cider vinegar. Just mix equal parts of apple cider vinegar and water and store in a container or a spray bottle. You can also add some essential oils or lemon juice to lessen the smell of the vinegar. Use cotton balls or spray it on your face.

43. REDUCE WRINKLES

Wrinkles are the hardest to prevent and diminish. Instead of spending so much money on lasers, pills and creams, try this natural homemade wrinkle-reducer solution brought to you by ACV. Apply this on your face regularly before going to bed and you'll start seeing positive changes after some time. Mix equal parts of apple cider vinegar and water and use a cotton ball to apply it on the face. Rinse with warm water and pat dry.

44. FACIAL WASH

Never again spend money on expensive facial wash that doesn't do much. Apple cider vinegar can also be used as a natural facial wash. Dilute 1 part apple cider vinegar in 2 parts water to reduce the effect of its acid content, but still be enough to get rid of bacteria. Apply the solution to your face and massage for a couple of minutes. Rinse after. Using apple cider as a facial wash will rid the skin of dead skin cells, bacteria and dirt.

45. ANTIFUNGAL

Fungal infections on the skin are quite common. This includes: athlete's foot, jock itch, ringworm, yeast infections, etc. The acetic acid in apple cider vinegar is well known for killing off living bacteria that cause these infections. It also prevents any more bacteria buildup on the skin for a maximum infection relief. Mix one part apple cider vinegar with 2 parts water. Soak a cotton ball into mixture and apply directly on the fungus-affected area. You can also choose to soak the skin area in the mixture directly for about 30 minutes or so.

46. SKIN WHITENING

We all want immaculate, rosy skin and try different products to achieve this—but most of them do very little. Some can even damage our skin if we're not careful! Using apple cider vinegar as a natural skin whitening ingredient will not only whiten skin but also leave it smooth and bacteria-free. Add apple cider vinegar to your bath and soak for 30 minutes at most.

47. MAKE HAIR DYE LAST LONGER

It is expensive to have one's hair dyed at a salon. That is why many chose to do it themselves at home. Even when the packet or packaging says a certain hair dye is permanent, it mostly is not true and will fade after a couple of weeks or months of shampooing and washing hair. To make your hair dye last longer, add apple cider vinegar to your next hair dye mixture.

48. GETS RID OF DANDRUFF

Dandruff comes from excess shampoo that attaches on the scalp and eventually becomes a sort-of-fungal infection. It is really hard to completely get rid of dandruff since it depends upon what your skin likes or dislikes when it comes to hygiene products sold in the market. Well, luckily, there is a homemade remedy for this. Mix apple cider vinegar with equal parts of water and store in a spray bottle. Spray on hair and leave for 30-60 minutes. Wash right after. The acid in apple cider vinegar will kill bacteria, prevent shampoo buildup and promote better scalp condition.

49. CLEARS ACNE

There are a lot of acne treatments out there and most of these formulas prove to be harmful to the skin rather than helpful. Therefore it is suggested to switch to the more natural way of treating any skin problems with ingredients found at home. Apple cider vinegar kills bacteria, eliminates excess oil, dirt and makeup and removes dead skin cells for a clearer skin. There are many ways and you can experiment and incorporate other ingredients to making this face mask but here are the basics that you must include:

- 1 tbsp apple cider vinegar

- 3 tbsp honey

- 1 cup warm water

Mix the ingredients in a bowl. Massage the mixture on face and let sit for 20 minutes. Rinse face with water and pat dry. You can also add green tea which will help in reducing skin inflammation and also kills bacteria.

50. WHITEN TEETH

Baking soda and apple cider vinegar makes a good combination for removing surface stains from teeth, making it whiter and brighter. Mix two parts of apple cider vinegar and one part baking soda into a small amount of water. Stir well to make a fine paste and use this as your toothpaste. Make sure the water is of enough amount to make a paste. Brush the mixture into teeth and after, rinse with water. Incorporate this routine a few times a week. You can just also directly gargle with apple cider vinegar to remove teeth stains.

51. SHINY HAIR

Apple cider vinegar is known for its many benefits for the hair. If you have dry damaged hair, apple cider vinegar is the answer for you. Many have tried this and there are numerous tutorials online. Mix equal part of apple cider vinegar with water and apply evenly on hair. Make sure to massage it into the scalp for it to reach the roots. Leave it for a couple of minutes. Shampoo hair then rinse. Repeat this once a week or once a month depending on hair conditions.

52. HEAL DRY, CRACKED FEET

Cracked feet is not easy to heal. One can use petroleum jelly to soften the skin on the feet area, but a more efficient alternative is using apple cider vinegar. The acetic acid in apple cider vinegar helps soften the skin and makes exfoliation easier. Soak feet in a mixture of apple cider vinegar and water for 30 minutes and at least three to four times a week. It will also kill living bacteria and eliminates odor. Plus soaking feet in the water is refreshing and relaxing.

53. REMOVES SKIN TAGS

Skin tags are unwanted excess skin and flesh hanging in small blobs and may appear anywhere in the body, men and women alike. Besides alcohol and hydrogen peroxide, apple cider vinegar is also an effective agent for removing skin tags. First, wash the area with lukewarm water, apply anti-bacterial soap or solution and rinse well. Pour a small amount of apple cider vinegar on a cotton ball and squeeze out the excess. Apply on the area for a couple of minutes.

54. PREVENTS HAIR LOSS

Balding is treated in many different ways. There are a lot of natural remedies to hair loss and also in preventing them. Preventing and slowing down hair loss has never been easy until this. Apple cider vinegar can prevent hair loss with its pH balancing factor when applied on the scalp. Mix apple cider vinegar in equal part water. Massage on scalp right after shampooing. Rinse well to remove the smell and excess vinegar. Follow with a hair conditioner if desired.

55. GET RID OF VARICOSE VEINS

It is usually quite expensive to get varicose veins treated, but not anymore. Apple cider vinegar can help with diminishing their appearance. Apply undiluted apple cider vinegar to the skin over varicose veins and gently massage. Leave overnight and rinse the next morning. Make sure to apply a moisturizing lotion for the acid in apple cider may make skin dry.

56. DEFINES CURLS

The extent of up keep of curly hair is greater than that of straight hair. Curly hair goals are about defining those curls. Curly people don't want this curls fizzy and dry because that will cause hair to pop rather than hang down with volume. To condition your curls, use apple cider vinegar as your conditioner. Dilute 1/3 vinegar with 2/3 water and add essential oils and store in a spray bottle or any container. Apply this to hair after shampooing. Use two to three times a week or less as you please. Soft, voluminous, defined curly hair has never been this easy.

57. REDUCES FRIZZ

Getting rid of frizzy hair is tough especially in very humid or dry weather. Basking under the sun won't also help for it will leave hair dry and unnourished. To get tame frizzy hair, use apple cider vinegar as a conditioner. The acid in apple cider vinegar will help remove dirt and grease from hair. It also closes and covers hair cuticles resulting in smoother hair. Mix ½ cup of apple cider vinegar in a cup of warm water and apply to hair starting from the roots going all the way to the tips. Do this after shampooing and let it sit for a minute or so before rinsing.

58. RELAXING DETOX BATH

The smell may be strong but the benefits it gives to the body are numerous. Using apple cider vinegar as a detox bath will not only be relaxing but also fights a number of skin infections. It soothes sunburns, eliminates body odor, promotes healthy hair, and relieves joint pain. Simply fill up a bath tub with water and add 1-2 cups of apple cider vinegar. Soak for 20-30 minutes and make sure to wet your hair as well. Soak a washcloth in the mixture and gently apply on face. Take a shower after to get rid of the remaining vinegar water. You can also opt to add essential oils, coconut oil, lemon juice and fragrance.

59. REDUCE STRETCHMARKS

Stretchmarks are vein-like lines on areas where the skin was once stretched. While it is a fact that one should be proud of stretchmarks for they may have battled with reducing weight or pregnancy, there are people who would like to lighten them a bit. To diminish stretchmarks using apple cider vinegar you need the following:

- 1/2 cup apple cider vinegar

- 1 cup water

- Spray bottle

Fill the spray bottle with apple cider vinegar and water. Spray this mixture on the stretchmarks every night and leave it on. Wash it off the next morning and use a moisturizing soap or apply moisturizing lotion after because apple cider vinegar may make the skin dry. Repeat this routine daily until stretchmarks are completely erased.

60. STRENGTHEN NAILS

Weak, brittle nails are a hassle. It's quite frustrating trying to achieve that perfect long nail shape while having weak and brittle-prone finger nails. Apple cider vinegar can improve blood circulation under the fingernail area and keep nails moisturized. Mix a cup of apple cider vinegar. Soak fingers in the solution for 10 minutes or so before going to bed. You can also add a cup of beer, and 1/2 cup olive oil as you prefer. Beer, like apple cider vinegar, contains several minerals which are effective in nourishing and strengthening nails.

61. REMOVE BLACK HEADS

Black heads are caused by hair follicles that get clogged with dead skin cells, dirt, excess sebum and other impurities. It appears as small black and yellow bumps that are a hassle to get rid of and has a tendency to reappear again. The anti-bacterial and antiseptic properties in apple cider vinegar will eliminate bacteria and prevent further buildup in the skin pores. Mix equal parts apple cider vinegar and water and apply on blackheads using a cotton ball. Apply during nighttime before going to bed and rinse the areas in the morning.

62. IMPROVED HAIR GROWTH

With the many uses and exemplary benefits of apple cider vinegar when applied to hair, it can also improve hair growth and lessen hair loss. Apple cider vinegar stimulates better blood circulation in hair follicles. This is essential for encouraging hair growth and preventing hair loss. Also, blood carries nutrients to hair follicles which aid in strengthening hair roots and promoting growth. Blend a cup of water with four tablespoons of apple cider vinegar in a bowl or container. After shampooing, apply the mixture starting from the scalp, hair roots and running down the entire length of hair. Massage for two minutes then rinse.

63. NATURAL AFTERSHAVE

For those who have sensitive skin, hair removal is always an issue. Razor burn is the enemy of every man and woman. Use apple cider vinegar as an aftershave to disinfect and naturally heal razor burns. You'll need apple cider vinegar and cotton balls. After hair removal, simply pour apple cider vinegar in a cotton ball and apply to areas where needed. Take precaution since you are applying a highly acidic formula onto irritated skin.

64. REMOVES BAD BREATH

Bad breath is caused by bacteria in the mouth that doesn't seem to go away even by brushing tooth and gargling mouthwash. Apple cider vinegar can help with that. The acid in apple cider vinegar is great for removing bacteria and preventing its build up. To get rid of bad breath, first use baking soda to brush your teeth and rinse it off with water. You can opt to add baking soda to your toothpaste as you please. Next, take apple cider vinegar and rinse mouth then, lastly, rinse with water.

65. ELIMINATE FOOT ODOR

Apple cider vinegar is a natural deodorant. However, foot smell is relatively different from other bodily odor. To get rid of foot odor, xix 1 pat apple cider vinegar with 2 part water and soak feet in this mixture for about 20-30 minutes. You can also massage your feet while soaking it and add essential oils or lemon juice for a touch of fresh scent.

66. MASSAGE TREATMENT

After a heavy and stressful day, it is better just to lie down and relax. Make relaxing better with an apple cider vinegar hand and foot massage. Apple cider vinegar has many properties that soothe the skin and by just applying it to the skin and rubbing gently, it will greatly smoothen skin and relieve it of stress. You can also opt to add salt or sugar to form a scrub and that effectively get rid of dead skin cells. Or add fragrance for a fresh scent to calm the mind.

67. Dishes Detergent

Apple cider vinegar also proves to be an effective household cleaning agent when it comes to getting rid of stains, odor and bacteria. We don't want to sacrifice health just because of a small stain from a used plate. There also may be bacteria left, that can't be seen by the naked eye. Apple cider may help remove any remaining unwanted bacteria and germs from all kitchen utensils with just these things found in your kitchen counter. All you need is a jar, a dishwashing liquid, apple cider vinegar, and a sponge to remove stains, odor and bacteria from plates, mugs and other kitchen utensils. Simply mix apple cider vinegar with dishwashing liquid and use this to clean dishes.

68. CLEANS JEWELRY

There are numerous ways on how to clean off tarnish from jewelry. Several homemade cleaning solutions can be found on the internet with ingredients that can be found right in our kitchen. Apple cider vinegar proves to be a great agent in cleaning jewelry with its acetic acid content. Soak silver jewelry in a mixture of ½ cup apple cider vinegar and 2 tablespoons of baking soda for an hour and the results will be surprising. You can also opt to just soak jewelry in apple cider vinegar for 10-15 minutes and occasionally brush the jewelry using a toothbrush to get rid of tarnish and dirt.

69. DEODORIZE REFRIGERATOR

The smell of rotten meat, fish and vegetables in refrigerators cannot be avoided. A lot of people follow different ways when it comes to getting rid of that odor, like cleaning it with lemon or baking soda. Another technique would be to clean it with apple cider vinegar. The acid in ACV can get rid of unwanted bacteria and pungent odor in your refrigerators. Since vinegar has a very peculiar smell, it is advised to use just a small amount; half a glass would be enough for a medium-sized fridge.

70. CLEANS TOOTHBRUSH

With all the other things that apple cider vinegar can cleanse, your toothbrush is also included among them. Continuous use of toothbrush for cleaning teeth and mouth will leave bacteria and germs to grow in your toothbrush. It is recommended to also clean your toothbrush to remove bacteria from it. Apple cider vinegar is very effective for dissolving germs and preventing bacteria buildup. Pour ½ cup of water into a glass. Add 2 tablespoons of apple cider vinegar and 2 tsp of baking soda. Use this to soak toothbrush for about 30 minutes to an hour.

71. PRESERVE THE COLOR OF CLOTHES

After wearing a shirt a couple of times, color fading is inevitable. Some people find themselves buying several pieces of the same shirt because its color fades with just several uses and washes. Letting clothes dry under the heat of the sun may also cause color fading on clothes. There are several ways on how to preserve clothes color with just natural ingredients found in our homes.

Baking soda, salt and pepper are just some. Apple cider vinegar also lessens the chances of color fading. Add apple cider vinegar while you're doing laundry and it will preserve clothes color. Don't worry, the vinegar won't leave the shirt smelling like salad dressing, the detergent will get rid of the smell.

72. SHINES WOOD FURNITURE

Wood furniture is a great accessory at home and it gives every home a touch of nature. While it adds beauty and is a plus in modern design, its upkeep is also a bit of a hassle. Constantly keeping wood floors and furniture shiny would hurt our pockets at the expense of buying those floor and furniture formulas. There is, however, a natural alternative for the up keep of wood furniture and floors and it all can be found in our homes.

- ½ cup apple cider vinegar

- ½ cup olive oil

- 20-30 drops lemon or orange oil

Mix all ingredients in a spray bottle and use to clean wood flooring and furniture. Continue use once a month for best results.

73. WHITENS LAUNDRY

White shirts, pants and underwear are essential and mostly the basic clothing that we should have in our wardrobes. But often these are the most impossible to wash; especially with the number of stains, dirt, sweat, etc. that has to be removed to restore its whiteness. Apple cider vinegar, with its dirt and stain-removing components, can help whiten laundry. Add a relatively ample amount of apple cider when doing laundry and it will immediately whiten your whitest clothes.

74. CLEAN AND DEODORIZE TOILET BOWL

A lot of cleaning solutions are out in the market. While most of them are effective in cleaning and deodorizing, the chemicals in these solutions may be harmful to human health. Most people opt to use natural solutions in cleaning toilets for it proves to be great for removing stains, dirt and bad odor. Apple cider vinegar with its acetic acid gets rid of bacteria and germ buildup in your toilet bowl and leaves it odor free. Mix apple cider vinegar and water in a spray bottle and use as toilet cleaner.

75. ACTS AS A FABRIC SOFTENER

Aside from apple cider vinegar preserving the color of clothes, it also softens fabrics. Apple cider vinegar acts as a fabric softener when added to your daily washing routine. Just add a cup or two of apple cider vinegar while the washing machine is running.

76. FERTILIZE PLANTS

Just like humans, plants may die out of excessive chemical exposure. While a lot of fertilizers out there are effective, spraying it on plants for human consumption could be harmful. Apple cider vinegar can be effectively used as an alternative fertilizer for plants without causing human harm.

Because apple cider is acidic, it is advised that you use it only on those plants which are acid friendly. Mix a cup of apple cider vinegar with water in a spray bottle and spray on to plants. Make sure to drown the apple cider vinegar with enough water so that it isn't too strong to harm the soil and plants.

77. HOMEMADE TOOTHPASTE

Using apple cider vinegar as a natural, homemade alternative for toothpaste will leave teeth whiter, mouth fresh and free from odor. Its acetic acid will kill living bacteria and prevent further buildup. You will need the following ingredients:

- 1/2 tablespoon apple cider vinegar

- 1 tablespoon baking soda

- Water

Mix all the ingredients. Make sure water is enough to make a paste. Use as alternative toothpaste 2-3 times a week or as needed.

78. ROOM FRESHENER

There are so many room air fresheners in the market mostly made from chemicals we are not aware of if any of these have harmful effects to the human body. It is always better to switch to the more natural solutions that are proven effective. Apple cider vinegar with its many home uses, can also be used as an air freshener. Dilute a cup of apple cider vinegar in 1 cup water and add to spray bottle. Spray around the room for a fresh, clean scent. You can also add lemon juice or fragrance to enhance the scent.

79. UNCLOG DRAINS

It's frustrating to have a clogged drain. It makes cooking and washing dishes harder than it should be. To unclog drain, first, pour ½ cup of baking soda down the drain. The baking soda will be good for making a reaction together with its bacteria-fighting agents. Then pour 2 cups of apple cider vinegar. The reaction will cause some bubbling that results from the chemical reaction. Leave it for at least five minutes then let tap water flow down the drain to rinse out any remaining solution. Repeat steps until the desired outcome is achieved.

80. USE AS A FLEA SPRAY

The longer the dog hair is, the more it is prone to fleas living in it. Apple cider vinegar is an effective alternative way to get rid of flea from dogs and other animals. Simply mix apple cider vinegar with water and place in a spray bottle. Spray on to pet dog and make sure to avoid any open wounds, ears, mouth and eyes. Wash with water when areas specified has direct contact with apple cider vinegar.

81. USE AS DOG SHAMPOO

Dogs are man's best friend. Therefore, we take care of them like how we usually take care of our fellow human beings. Vaccination, food, and other essential needs of dogs may be costly. You do not have to visit expensive stores for dog shampoos that cost a fortune. With this alternative dog shampoo, you only need a couple of ingredients found at home and is very easy to make and use.

- 2 cups warm water

- ½ cup apple cider vinegar

- ¼ liquid soap or baby shampoo

You can also add lemon for fragrance. Mix all the ingredients well in a bottle and apply on a dog during bath time.

82. ACV AS A FLY CATCHER

Fruit flies are annoyingly fast and nearly impossible to catch, much less get rid of them. Fight fruit flies with just simply 3 items found at home. All you need is a cup of apple cider vinegar, dish soap and a jar or a small wide-mouthed container. First and foremost toss out any overripe fruit. Pour both cup of apple cider vinegar and a couple of drops of dish soap into the jar. Mix the ingredients thoroughly. Place the trap in the area where the flies are and wait.

83. HOME WEED KILLER

Apple cider vinegar has been proved to be a helpful all around house cleaner. Clearing weeds is not an exception. With its acetic acid content, apple cider vinegar can kill unwanted weeds in your back yard. Just gather these ingredients and follow the steps:

- 1 cup apple cider vinegar

- 1 teaspoon Epsom salt

- Spray bottle

Pour apple cider into your spray bottle then add the salt. Mix well until the salt is completely dissolved. Spray mixture to weeds. Apple cider vinegar may kill weeds and undesirable plants but it also has the ability to kill off those good and desirable plants. Always make sure you do not spray it on a plant you do want to keep.

84. DETER ANTS

Ants come from anywhere. One moment there are no sight of such and the next thing you'll find is them swarming left over food or any residue on the floor. Mix one part apple cider vinegar and one part water in a spray bottle. Ants follow one another in a trail going back and forth their colony, so spray the mixture along the ant trail. The smell will drive ants away.

85. AIR HUMIDIFIER

Air humidifiers are small machines use for putting moisture in room air to relive some health issues. Adding apple cider vinegar to your humidifier can reduce or eliminate bacteria growth in your homes that may cause health problems. Apple cider vinegar is also an effective way to disinfect and cleanse air humidifier machines.

86. CLEAN DOG'S EARS

You don't have to go to a pet salon and pay for an easy task you can do at home with just some ingredients found in the kitchen. Cleaning dog's ears may be tricky, but apple cider vinegar may just do the magic for you. Mix equal parts of apple cider vinegar and distilled water into a bowl.

Using a syringe or a dropper, carefully put 10 drops of the mixture into your dog's ears. Gently rub or massage the part near the ear in a circular motion then remove a hand to let the dog shake its head. You can also use cotton balls for checking your dog of any earwax and soak cotton ball onto the mixture to get rid of the wax.

87. USE AS MARINADE

Naturally, apple cider vinegar is used for cooking. Since apple cider vinegar can preserve the freshness and improve food taste, it is widely used in many food recipes in different ways. Aside from its many uses, apple cider vinegar is an essential ingredient in making your fish or chicken marinade. Here is a marinade recipe you can try at home:

- 2 cups apple cider vinegar

- ½ cup olive oil

- 2 teaspoons jalapeno pepper sauce

- 2 teaspoons cayenne pepper

- 2 tablespoons soy sauce

- 1 teaspoon salt

- 1/2 teaspoon garlic powder

88. WASH FRUIT AND VEGETABLES

Most fruits and vegetables carry with them bacteria and other harmful chemicals from fertilizers. Consumption of these would greatly affect health. That's why growing your own vegetables and fruit garden is advisable. But for those who still buy vegetables and fruits at grocery stores, make sure to get rid of any harmful toxins from your produce. Mix equal parts of apple cider and water and store it in a spray bottle. Spray this to your produce and leave for about 5 minutes before rinsing again. The acetic acid in apple cider vinegar will help get rid of harmful toxins. You can also just use apple cider vinegar as a rinse. It will leave your produce fresh too.

89. BOIL EGGS BETTER

Notice how susceptible to breaking some eggs can be when you boil them? The acid in apple cider vinegar creates a chemical reaction that keeps eggs from cracking during boiling. If it happens that there are cracks, apple cider vinegar will thicken the egg white and prevent it from spilling further. Simply do the same routine for boiling eggs but add 1/2 cup of apple cider vinegar. You will have perfect hard boiled eggs in no time!

90. PRESERVE FOOD

Always keeping your food refrigerated may take away its freshness eventually. The great news is that apple cider vinegar can also be used as a food preserver and help it stay fresh without keeping it refrigerated for longer periods. Apple cider vinegar has a mellow aroma compared to white vinegar, and a tart acid flavor so it does not affect fruit and vegetable colors. Apple cider juice is also a great option for pickles as it has a fruity flavor that blends well with spices. It is also good for cucumbers and peeled apples. Simply soak vegetables and fruits in apple cider vinegar to improve food taste and keep it fresh.

91. MAKE BUTTERMILK

Reluctant to buy a whole carton of buttermilk when you only need one cup? Apple cider vinegar is a good substitute for making buttermilk. You can make any of the following alternatives to making buttermilk: 1 cup of soy milk and add 1 tbsp of apple cider vinegar, 1 cup almond milk and 1 tbsp of apple cider vinegar, or 1cup coconut milk and 1 tbsp of apple cider vinegar. Let it sit for 5-15 minutes until the mixture starts to thicken. Use these for making pancakes and waffles or as an ingredient to making cakes.

92. SAUCE

Apple cider vinegar is a natural home cooking ingredient and is an alternative to a lot of cooking needs. Using apple cider vinegar as a sauce will greatly increase food taste and it is good for one's health too. It can be used solely or added with other ingredients to make a sauce. Use any of these seasonings to add to apple cider vinegar to make the best sauces: olive oil, Dijon mustard, garlic, sea salt, pepper, lemon juice, honey, etc.

93. TENDERIZE MEAT

There are just as many tenderizers to prepare meat out there and mostly online as there is so many ways to cook meat. Tenderizing meat will make it soft and easy to cook. Soak meat in apple cider vinegar to tenderize it and prepare it for cooking. Add a couple of spices to create a marinade and greatly help with meat taste. Using apple cider vinegar to tenderize meat will not only make it easy to cook but also leaves a sweet taste to the meat.

94. SALAD DRESSING

Apple cider vinegar is most commonly used as a food seasoning. By adding apple cider vinegar to your next salad dressing, your recipe will have that enough sour taste to please your taste buds. There are a lot of ways to create your salad dressing with ACV, below is one:

- 1/2 cup apple cider vinegar

- 1/2 cup olive oil

- 2tbs honey or pure maple syrup

- 1 lemon juice

- 1/2 teaspoon basil, parsley, and/or oregano

95. ENHANCE SOUP TASTE

The many cooking uses for apple cider vinegar proves it to be a top and essential ingredient in the kitchen. One can tell when soup has apple cider in it or not with the taste apple cider creates. Add a tablespoon or two of apple cider vinegar on your next soup to enhance its taste. Its numerous health benefits is already a plus for using it as an ingredient in home recipes.

96. COCKTAILS

While all the many uses of apple cider vinegar, it is great as an addition to food and beverages. Apple cider vinegar contains alcohol, which is in fact, a great mix to your cocktails. Here is a cocktail recipe with apple cider vinegar you can try at home:

- Cider and Pomegranate Margarita

- 4 oz apple cider vinegar

- 2 oz pomegranate juice

- 2 oz tequila

- ½ oz fresh lime juice

- ½ oz simple syrup

- Coarse salt

Add a slice of lemon or lime on top and a stick umbrella to complete the cocktail drink. Enjoy.

97. LEMON SUBSTITUTE

Apple cider vinegar like a lemon has acidic properties that make recipes tastier. Should you ever run out of lemon at home, you can use apple cider vinegar as a substitute.

98. HEALTHY ADDITION TO YOUR MORNING SMOOTHIE

Smoothies are an option to eating healthy with the addition of more palatable ingredients like milk, honey, yogurt, ice cream, cookies and fruits. Smoothies also increase energy and are consumed widely by people before or after their daily workouts and exercise. Aside from drinking your daily dose of apple cider vinegar to regulate natural body pH, boost immune system and metabolism and all the other benefits, you can just add ACV on your next smoothie and eventually get all the health benefits stated. It adds a sweet taste to the smoothie too.

99. ADD TO YOUR TEA

Apple cider vinegar is proven to have detoxifying properties. While it can be added to water, it is much better added to tea. With addition to any of the following: honey, cinnamon or lemon juice, tea will be perfect for a rainy day spent indoors.

100. BONE BROTH

Bone broth has the following benefits to the body: supports proper adrenal function, strengthens the immune system, Alkalizes body, mineralize the body and strengthening the bones. Apple cider vinegar, when added to bone broth, acts as a solvent that helps pull calcium and other minerals from the bone while it slowly simmers. This increases the amount of calcium and mineral content in bone broth and makes it more nutritious than ever. The goal is to extract as abundant as minerals and nutrients as possible from the bones.

So there you have it, a hundred different uses for apple cider vinegar—from health problems to everyday home cooking, you're sure to benefit from a single bottle of it.